NAT

# Nature's Colour Codes

N H Hawes

Hammersmith Health Books
London, UK

First published in 2017 by Hammersmith Health Books – an imprint of
Hammersmith Books Limited
4/4A Bloomsbury Square, London WC1A 2RP, UK
www.hammersmithbooks.co.uk

**Note**: No book can replace the diagnostic expertise and medical advice
of a trusted physician. Please be certain to consult your doctor before making any
decisions that affect your health or extreme changes to your diet, particularly if
you suffer from any medical condition or have any symptom that may require
treatment. Whilst the advice and information in this book are believed to be true
and accurate at the date of going to press, neither the author nor the publisher
can accept any legal responsibility or liability for any errors or omissions that
may have been made.

British Library Cataloguing in Publication Data: A CIP record of this book is
available from the British Library.

ISBN (print edition): 978-1-78161-087-9
ISBN (ebook): 978-1-78161-088-6

Commissioning editor: Georgina Bentliff
Cover design by: Julie Bennett, Bespoke Publishing Ltd
Typeset by: Julie Bennett, Bespoke Publishing Ltd
Production: Helen Whitehorn, Path Projects Ltd
Printed and bound by TJ International Ltd

# Contents

# About Nature Cures

This pocketbook is a guide to natural ways to treat health issues. The information is drawn from my website www.naturecures.co.uk and my comprehensive book *Nature Cures: The A to Z of Ailments and Natural Foods*, available from www.hammersmithbooks. co.uk. For more detail about the nutrients and foods listed in this pocketbook, please do refer to these sources.

In both this book and my comprehensive works the sources of the information I've used are too numerous to list without at least doubling the size; if there is any fact or recommendation that is of concern, please do contact me via www.naturecures.co.uk.

This pocketbook represents a compilation of years of research but is no substitute for visiting a qualified health practitioner so please do consult such, especially your doctor with regard to any prescription medications, before making signficant changes to your diet, lifestyle or health regime.

## *Other titles in the series include*

*Let Roots Be Your Medicine*
*Grow Your Own Health Garden*
*Air-purifying House Plants*
*Recovery from Injury, Surgery and Infection*

# Introduction

In this little book I explain why it is so important to eat not just a good quantity of fresh vegetables and fruit every day ('five a day' plus) but as wide a variety as possible in terms of type and of *colour*. As you will find out, each of the colours is produced by different phytochemicals that are essential for good health. What we know is summarised below, but there is of course a great deal more we do not yet know, which is why *Nature Cures* is all about consuming whole foods, not isolated nutrients or supplements, provided these are fresh and, if at all possible, organic. (Organic foods may be more expensive, but they are much more nutrient-dense so you do not need to eat as much to get the nutrients you require while avoiding the chemicals non-organic farming involves.)

Nature has kindly colour-coded foods for us and each colour is associated with different compounds that the body needs on a regular, and often daily, basis. Eating five of just one colour per day can leave us deficient in the vital nutrients of the other colours – we need to 'eat the rainbow' (see page 10). There are over 100 minerals and many thousands of other types of nutrients which work with each other (as 'co-factors') at a molecular level. Exactly what works with what, when and why is the subject of ongoing research; it will be many years before we understand this in all its complexity.

Artificially coloured foods confuse the picture. Not only do they suggest nutrients are present when they are not, but the food dyes concerned have been associated with many physical and mental health problems, especially in children, the elderly and those with allergies or a weakened immune system. (For a full list see pages 53-82.) A key message of *Nature Cures* is 'Always read the label for the list of ingredients'. If you are not used to doing this you will be amazed by what you find.

## *A note about genetically modified foods*

Foods that have been genetically modified may not contain the nutrients associated with natural food colours described in this book. The purpose of genetic modification is generally not to increase nutrient levels but to increase yield and lessen wastage. (Interestingly, research has shown that animals will avoid genetically modified foods, when given a choice; it appears they instinctively know which foods are more likely to provide them with the nutrients they require. Humans seem to have lost this ability.)

Foods are often genetically modified to withstand more powerful pesticides, herbicides and fungicides. This means that more of these chemicals can be used without destroying the crops but humans end up ingesting traces of ever-increasingly powerful chemicals that may reach toxic levels as they build-up in the body's stores. Fungicides and pesticides may also upset the balance of micro-organisms in our gut that help us break down our food, leading to many serious health issues, allergies and nutrient deficiencies; the beneficial bacteria in the gut are protective and also help to manufacture many vital nutrients, such as short-chain fatty acids (a source of energy) and vitamin K2 that directs calcium to our bones.

The *Nature Cures* advice is to avoid GM foods when following Nature's Colour Codes.

## *A note about food production and nutrient deficiencies*

*Nature Cures* focuses on the healing and health-giving properties of natural foods. However, in modern times we have the problem that our fruit and vegetables have less nutritional content than they did even 10 years ago. This is the result of changes in both farming methods (to increase yield) and food production (to increase 'shelf life'). For example, shelf life can be increased by stripping the more perishable but nutritionally important components from grains (e.g. wheat germ), and then adding back cheaper or artificial versions of the nutrients lost. Often the substances used for this 'fortification' are inferior to the original and if relied upon can lead to nutrient deficiencies.

For instance, the type of vitamin D that humans can absorb is vitamin D3 but often, it is vitamin D2, which is not easily absorbed, that is added to foods and sold as a supplement. Meanwhile, there is little awareness that vitamin K2 is needed as a co-factor for vitamin D.

Vitamin B2 (riboflavin) is very difficult to add to foods and is destroyed by light so when labels on breakfast cereals say there is 'added riboflavin' it does not mean that you will actually be absorbing enough of it on a daily basis from cereals alone.

When the body is nutritionally deficient it cannot work optimally or protect itself against infection, or the effects of long-term stress.

Everybody is unique and, as the old saying goes, 'one man's poison may be another man's medicine'; this is why it is so difficult to establish the exact reasons behind what causes disease and ill health, or good health and longevity. However, it should always be remembered that naturally colourful whole foods do no harm, unless there are specific intolerances to a certain food group, such as the nightshade family, and most provide a multitude of beneficial nutrients whereas drugs, supplements and refined and processed foods with artificial additives can cause nutritional imbalances and deficiencies that may lead to illness or uncomfortable, and sometimes seriously debilitating, side-effects.

## The importance of minerals in the diet

The most powerful way of building health is on a firm foundation made up of the basic elements beneath our feet. These basic elements are the many minerals and trace elements that make up the earth's crust and are also present within the human body.

Natural unrefined sea salt contains these minerals in abundance – 92 have been identified. Of these, 24 have been proven essential for the maintenance of good health; the contribution of others is being discovered by scientists all the time. Unfortunately, most sea salt is refined and bleached before turning up in the supermarket or health food store, leaving just two elements (sodium and chorine combined to become sodium chloride) which provide the salt-taste we increasingly crave. Other elements, such as calcium, magnesium, potassium and iodine, are removed and sold separately to industry. We may even find we are buying them back at greatly enhanced prices in the form of mineral supplements!

Only traces of many minerals are required by the body, but due to today's intense farming techniques much of the mineral content has been lost from the soil. Minerals are absolutely vital for many cellular processes. Although the body can store minerals, it cannot manufacture them so consuming a wide range of natural foods can help replenish stores that are used up or lost.

This is as important for those who are unwell or taking medications as it is for those that do strenuous exercise or sports. Minerals are lost through perspiration, and many drugs (including alcohol) block the absorption of minerals or cause the body to lose them in the urine. For example, alcohol causes the body to expel zinc in this way.

An imbalance between vitamin C and vitamin E can also cause mineral imbalances. Vitamin C increases iron uptake, which vitamin E inhibits and vitamin C lowers manganese and zinc, while vitamin E helps increase manganese and zinc absorption. Therefore, balanced amounts of both are required to maintain a steady ratio. Always consuming vitamin C-rich fruit with vitamin E-rich nuts or seeds is one way to maintain this balance.

All vegetables and fruits begin to deteriorate nutritionally as soon as you cut through the protective outer skin which means that most pre-made store-bought juices and pre-prepared and packaged chopped fruits and vegetables are of less value nutritionally; most also contain added sugar, artificial sweeteners and other artificial ingredients to preserve or colour them – again, read the labels!

There is one exception to the above which is foods from the *allium* family (onions, garlic etc). Allicin is a powerful antibacterial, antifungal and anti-parasitic compound that protects plants from microbes and is beneficial in many ways to human health but it is not present in these foods in their natural state. When they are chopped or otherwise damaged, the enzyme alliinase in them acts on the chemical alliin, converting it into allicin. It is therefore important to chop foods that produce allicin, such as chives, garlic, leeks and onions, then set them aside for 10 minutes for this process to take place, before cooking or consuming them.

# Why we should 'eat the rainbow'

Nature's colours give strong clues about the nutrient content of foods which we should not ignore. For instance; beetroots are rich in betacyanins and iron which gives them their deep red colour and provides the essential ingredients for optimum health. Iron is essential to the production of red blood cells that carry vital oxygen to all parts of the body and betacyanins have a whole host of amazing health benefits that are listed on page 23.

Some vegetables contain more than one colour. For instance, spring onions have green leaves and white roots. This means there are the nutrients associated with both these colours present so the whole of the plant should be eaten and will provide the nutrients listed for green and white below. The same goes for beetroot and beetroot leaves and turnips and their leaves.

Some vegetables, fruits and nuts contain different healthy nutrients in both their flesh and skins so both should be consumed. Apples, aubergines, potatoes and sweet potatoes are examples. Orange, lime and lemon peel has powerful antioxidant properties and can help to protect the brain and heart and therefore should be included in the diet. Skins should only ever be discarded if they are completely inedible, such as those of bananas, watermelons or pumpkins.

The colour of foods can also indicate the ripeness, which again has an impact on the nutritional content. For instance, green unripe bananas are richer in resistant starch and fibre than ripened yellow bananas while Japanese scientists have found that a fully ripe banana produces a substance called tumour necrosis factor (TNF). This compound has the ability to combat abnormal cells and protect against cancer. They discovered that as the banana ripens and develops dark brown and black spots and patches on its skin, the concentration of TNF increases. They say that the degree of anti-cancer effect corresponds to the degree of ripeness of the fruit.

## A note about 'free radicals' and 'anti-oxidants'

Throughout the descriptions of beneficial plant pigments below there are references to the importance of preventing 'free radical damage' with the aid of 'antioxidants'. They are therefore prefaced with the following explanation.

'Free radicals' and 'antioxidants' are terms used to explain intricate molecular processes which would take up too much space to explain fully in this pocket book but are described in depth on the Nature Cures 'Cleanse and Detoxify' page in the comprehensive volume *Nature Cures: The A to Z of Ailments and Natural Foods*.

Put simply, a free radical is a molecule that is missing an

electron. Because of this it is unstable and reactive and attacks other molecules to steal an electron in order to become stable again. But the molecule it steals the electron from then becomes a free radical itself and this causes a chain reaction, like a domino effect, which can lead to cell damage within the body.

Heavy metal molecules can greatly intensify this reaction, if they collide with free radicals, causing far greater damage, which may be one of the root causes of Alzheimer's and other brain degeneration diseases.

Many factors can induce free-radical formation in the environment. They cause clothes to fade, food to spoil, metal to rust, pipes to leak, plastics to deteriorate, paint to fade and peel and works of art to degrade.

In the human body, free radicals can be useful because they help important reactions to take place. They arise normally during metabolism and sometimes the immune system's white blood cells purposefully create them to neutralise bacteria and viruses. Free radicals are a natural by-product of the body when it turns food into energy and, normally, the body makes its own antioxidant enzymes to deal with them. Catalase, glutathione peroxidase and superoxide dismutase are three such enzymes and they require micronutrient cofactors such as copper, iron, manganese, selenium and zinc for their activity.

An excess of free radicals becomes a problem because they attack the body itself, damaging key cellular molecules, such as DNA (our genetic code). Cells with damaged DNA are more prone to developing cancer, and free-radical damage accumulates with age.

An antioxidant is not actually a substance; it is a behaviour. Any compound that can donate electrons to eliminate free radicals, without becoming a free radical itself, has antioxidant properties.

Some antioxidant molecules are too big to go through the gut wall so they work in the gut itself. Some antioxidants are water-soluble so can go where the fat-soluble ones cannot. Some work on the surface of cells and some work inside cells. Because different antioxidants work in different areas of the body, the key is to eat as wide a range of foods with antioxidant abilities as possible.

*Nutrients with antioxidant abilities*

- Alpha-carotene
- Alpha-lipoic acid
- Astaxanthin
- Beta-carotene
- Beta-cryptoxanthin
- Carnitine
- Catalase
- Catechins
- Coenzyme Q10
- Flavonoids
- Glutathione
- Iridium
- Lutein and zeaxanthin
- Lycopene
- Manganese
- Melatonin
- Phenols and polyphenols
- Phytoestrogens
- Quercetin

- Resveratrol
- Selenium
- Superoxide dismutase
- Uric acid
- Vitamin A
- Vitamin C
- Vitamin E

# The six colour categories of natural foods

Choose at least one small serving of each of the following six colour categories each day if you can. Make two of them fruit and four of them vegetables and at least one should be a leafy green.

- Green
- Orange/yellow
- Red
- Black/blue/purple/violet
- Cream/white
- Brown/gold

## 1. Green
**Chlorophyll** and **carotenoids** give the green pigment found in: apples, alfalfa, algae, artichoke (globe), ashitaba, asparagus, avocado, bell peppers, broad beans, broccoli, Brussel sprouts, cabbage, celery, chilli peppers, chives, chlorella, cress, courgettes, grapes, olives, herb leaves, kale, kiwi fruit, lettuce, lime and peel,

mung beans, okra, peas, pumpkin seeds, rhubarb, rocket, runner beans, seaweed, spinach, spirulina, spring onions, watercress, winged beans and sprouted seeds, grains, nuts and legumes.

## 2. Orange and yellow

**Curcumin** gives turmeric its yellow colour and **anthoxanthins, betaxanthins, carotenoids** and/or **chalcones** give the yellow and orange colours found in: apricots, bell peppers, butternut squash, carrots, chick peas, chilli peppers, corn, ginger, lemons, lentils, mango, oranges, papaya, peaches, pineapple, prickly pear, pumpkin, swede, sweet potato, tangerines, turmeric, the peel of yellow and orange citrus fruits and whole grains.

## 3. Red

**Anthoxanthins, betacyanins, carotenoids** and/or **lycopene** provide the red pigment in: apples, asparagus, bell peppers, cabbage (red), cherries, chilli peppers, cranberries, goji berries, grapefruit (pink), grapes (red and black), guava, oranges (blood), pears (red), mung beans, persimmons, pinto beans, prickly pear, radishes, raspberries, rhubarb, red chokeberry, kidney beans, onions (red), pomegranates, raspberries, rhubarb, rose hips, saw palmetto berries, strawberries, sumac, Swiss chard, tomatoes and watermelon.

**Astaxanthin** causes the pink/red colour in seafood, such as lobster, prawns, salmon and shrimp. The highest concentration is found in red krill oil. (Note that in farmed salmon the pink colour is produced by feeding them with lab-produced astaxanthin as they would otherwise be grey.)

## 4. Black, blue, purple and violet

**Anthocyanins** and **betacyanins** (never together) give the blue to black colours and are often most concentrated in the skins and/or stems of food crops such as: acai berry, purple aubergine, beetroot, bilberries, black bananas, black beans, blackberries, black chokeberry, black currants, black tea, blueberries, broccoli (purple variety), cherries, chokeberries, cranberries, dates, elderberry, figs, black grapes, black olives, kidney beans, maqui berries, mulberries, onions (red), navy beans, plums, poppy seeds, potatoes (red-skinned), prickly pear, prunes, purple broccoli tops, radishes, raisins, sweet potato (skins), Swiss chard and winged beans.

## 5. Cream and white

**Anthoxanthins** give the cream and white colours found in: white aubergine, just-ripe bananas, Brazil nuts, butter beans, cauliflower, celery, chestnuts, coconut, garlic, Jerusalem artichoke, leeks, macadamia nuts, mung beans, mushrooms, navy beans, onions, parsnip, peanuts, pecans, pine nuts, pistachios, potatoes, radishes, soya beans, spring onions and turnips.

### 6. Brown and gold

Brown and golden foods can contain a variety of the above pigment nutrients. Examples include: brown rice, cocoa beans, dates, mushrooms, nuts, potato skins, seeds and whole grains.

# The health benefits of the nutrients that colour foods

The following list of nutrients in foods, that produce their colours, is by no means complete as more are being discovered all the time. However, it provides the reader with some reasons why the consumption of colourful foods is vital for ultimate health.

## Anthocyanins (blue to black)

The term anthocyanin was initially coined to indicate the substance responsible for the colour of cornflowers and derives from the Greek term *anthos* 'flower' and *kuanos* 'blue' and refers to a group of water-soluble polyphenols that are responsible for the black, blue, lilac, mauve, pink, purple, red or violet colour of many flowers, fruits and vegetables.

Anthocyanins are a water-soluble bioflavonoid pigment and the colour will depend on the pH of the solution they are in. They are red when the pH is below three (highly acid), blue at pH higher than 11 (very alkali) and violet at neutral pH 7. Bioflavonoids are produced by plants for self-protection against sun, irradiation, diseases and biological enemies. With the harsh cold weather and high solar radiation in Chile, these factors guaranteed particularly high anthocyanins in the fruits and berries that grow in that region.

Some of the most colourful foods contain these bioflavonoids which are best known for their powerful antioxidant properties and healing power inside the body. They have been found to help slow down age-related motor changes, such as those seen in Alzheimer's or Parkinson's disease, prevent the oxidisation of certain compounds and fight attacks on the body from harmful chemicals. The many health benefits of anthocyanins include anti-carcinogen qualities and improved heart health.

They also increase vitamin C levels within cells, decrease the breakage of small blood vessels, protect against free-radical damage and help prevent destruction of collagen - the connective tissue under the skin - by helping the collagen fibres link together in a way that strengthens the connective tissue matrix. They also reduce blood glucose levels and improve insulin sensitivity due to the reduction of retinol-binding-protein-4 so are useful in preventing diabetes and can help with treating obesity.

'Myocardial ischaemia' means there is a reduced blood supply and therefore oxygen to the heart muscle, usually due to atherosclerosis of the coronary arteries. Its risk increases with age, diabetes, high blood pressure, high LDL cholesterol levels and smoking. When blood supply is restored, after a period of ischaemia (this is called 'reperfusion'), injury to the tissues can occur. Bioflavonoids such as the anthocyanins can reduce oxidative damage to organ cells during this process.

*Types of anthocyanins*

- Apigeninidin
- Aurantinidin
- Capensinidin
- Cyanidin
- Delphinidin
- Europinidin
- Hirsutidin
- Luteolinidin
- Malvidin
- Pelargonidin
- Peonidin
- Petunidin
- Pulchellidin
- Rosinidin
- Tricetinidin

Malvidin, in conjunction with chlorogenic acid and pelargonidin chloride, is a critical cofactor in the anti-proliferative defence against colon cancer and liver cancer cells, but without the other two cofactors (chlorogenic acid and pelargonidin chloride) the process will not take place. Malvidin is cytotoxic to human leukaemia cells by stopping the cancer cell cycle and inducing apoptosis (cell suicide).

Any illness that ends with '-itis' is an inflammatory one. Anthocyanins exhibit powerful anti-inflammatory activity and do it as well as drugs for the same purposes, without the negative side effects.

*Other health benefits of anthocyanins*

- Improve eyesight.
- Maintain small blood vessel integrity by stabilising capillary walls and increasing capillary permeability.
- Neutralise enzymes that destroy connective tissue, prevent oxidants from damaging connective tissue and repair damaged proteins in the blood-vessel walls.
- Promote cardiovascular health by preventing oxidation of low-density lipoproteins (LDL) and protecting blood vessel walls from oxidative damage.
- Reduce allergic reactions.
- Support healthy blood sugar levels.

Natural sources of anthocyanins are: acai berry, apples (red), aubergine, beans (black and red), beetroot, bilberries, blackberries, black currants, black rice, blueberries, broccoli tops (purple), cabbage (red), cashew nuts, cherries, chokeberries, cranberries, elderberry, grapefruit (pink), grapes (red and black), kidney beans, maqui berries, mulberries, onions (red), oranges (blood), pears (red), plums, potatoes (red skinned), pomegranates, radishes (red), raspberries, rhubarb, rosehips, saw palmetto berries, strawberries, sumac, sweet potato (purple variety), Swiss chard and winged beans.

**NOTE**: Anthocyanins are mostly concentrated in the skins of fruits and vegetables.

### *Anthoxanthins (cream and white)*

Anthoxanthins are water-soluble pigments which range from white or colourless to a creamy yellow and red, often in the petals of flowers. These pigments are generally whiter in an acid medium and yellower in an alkaline medium. Consuming foods rich in anthoxanthins has been found to reduce stroke risk, promote heart health, prevent cancer and reduce inflammation.

- Those undergoing treatment for complex corneal diseases, whose underlying eye health condition is caused or aggravated by inflammation, might find increased symptom relief by including more anthoxanthin-rich foods in their diets.
- Natural sources of anthoxanthins are bananas (just ripe), butter beans, butternut squash, cauliflower, celery, chestnuts, coconut, garlic, Jerusalem artichoke, leeks, macadamia nuts, mung beans, mushrooms, navy beans, nuts, onions, parsnip, pine nuts, potatoes, radishes, soya beans, spring onions and turnips.

### *Astaxanthin (red)*

Astaxanthin is the most powerful antioxidant known to man and is capable of crossing the blood/brain barrier to protect the brain cells from free radicals. It also increases the activity of the liver enzymes that detoxify carcinogens and stimulates and enhances the immune system. Red krill oil is the highest source of this nutrient although it is also in other red and pink sea creatures such as crabs, lobsters, prawns and shrimp.

## Betalains (orange and yellow and blue to black)

The name 'betalain' comes from the Latin name of the common beetroot *Beta vulgaris*. Betalains are found in the petals of flowers, but may colour the fruits, leaves, stems and roots of plants that contain them. Betalains are aromatic indole derivatives synthesised from the amino acid (building block of proteins) tyrosine. There are two categories:

- **Betacyanins** are the red to violet pigments. Among the betacyanins present in plants are betanin, isobetanin, probetanin, and neobetanin.
- **Betaxanthins** are yellow to orange pigments. The betaxanthins present in plants include vulgaxanthin, miraxanthin, portulaxanthin, and indicaxanthin.

Where betalains occur in plants, they sometimes coexist with anthoxanthins (yellow to orange flavonoids, page 21), but never coincide with anthocyanins (blue to purple and black flavonoids). The betalains provide a higher antioxidant value than most other vegetables containing beta-carotene and have anti-inflammatory, anti-cancer and detoxifying properties and support the making of red blood cells.

- Natural sources of the betacyanins are: amaranth, apples, apricots, artichoke, beetroot (purple), broccoli (purple top),

cactus and whole grains.
- Natural sources of betaxanthins are: basidiomycota mushrooms, beetroot (golden), cucumber, prickly pear and Swiss chard.

*Health benefits of betacyanins*
- Stop the spread of cancerous tumours
- Prevent diseases of liver, kidney and pancreas
- Help reduce ulcers in the stomach
- Strengthen the lungs and immune system
- Improve vision and are good for treating eye redness
- Reduce pain after intense physical training and also menstrual pain
- Eliminate hard stools and prevent constipation
- Positively affect the colon
- Regulate high blood pressure
- Eliminate bad breath
- Help to treat acne and create healthy skin.

*Health benefits of betaxanthins*
- Can cross the blood-brain, -eye and -spinal barriers to help arrest free-radical damage in cell membranes, mitochondria and DNA
- Enhance immune cell strength and antibody activity
- Improve gastrointestinal health
- Improve cognitive function

- Help to maintain peak performance in athletes
- Protect the heart.

### Carotenoids (deep green, yellow, orange and red)

The name 'carotene' comes from the Latin 'carota' (carrot). The carotenoids are a group of more than 700 fat-soluble nutrients. Many are proving to be very important for health. They are categorised as either **xanthophylls** or **carotenes** according to their chemical composition. These compounds have the ability to inhibit the growth of many pre-cancerous tumours.

- Carotenoids act as antioxidants, meaning they tackle harmful free radicals that damage tissues throughout the body. The types of carotenoids that have other health benefits include alphacarotene, betacarotene and cryptoxanthin. The body can convert all of these to **vitamin A**. This vitamin helps keep the immune system working properly and it is needed for eye health. Yellow and orange foods like pumpkins and carrots are good sources of alpha- and betacarotene. These also contain betacryptoxanthin, as do sweet red bell peppers.

- Other types of carotenoids are **lutein** and **zeaxanthin** that occur naturally in the plant pigments of dark green leaves and, when consumed regularly, protect the retina from damage caused by the sun's harmful ultraviolet (UV) rays and high-energy visible (HEV) light. Prolonged exposure to UV and HEV rays may damage the retina and increase the risk of developing macular degeneration. Zeaxanthin is an important dietary carotenoid that is selectively absorbed into the retinal macula lutea (at the back of the inside of the eye), where it is thought to provide antioxidant and protective light-filtering functions which is how it offers protection against macular degeneration, especially in the elderly. Lutein and zeaxanthin can also reduce the risk of cataracts later in life.

- These antioxidants also have the ability to protect cells and other structures in the body from the harmful effects of free radicals.
- Lutein can also help to reduce the risk of breast cancer and heart disease and supports healthy skin, tissue, blood and the immune system.
- Natural sources of lutein and zeaxanthin are: apples, apricots, artichoke, asparagus, avocado, bell peppers, broccoli, Brussels sprouts, buckwheat, butternut squash, cantaloupe, caraway seeds, carrots, cherries, chlorella, chokeberries, corn, courgette, cress, cucumber, curry leaf, dandelion leaves, dates, eggs, garden peas (raw), green beans, kale, lettuce (romaine), mulberries, nectarines, peas, pistachio nuts, rye, spinach, sweet potato, tomatoes and watercress (raw).

**Lycopene** is the bright red carotenoid that is found in fruits and vegetables. It does not convert to vitamin A, but has important cancer-fighting properties and other health benefits. While it is not a vitamin, it is a powerful antioxidant. Consuming lycopene regularly helps to reduce the risk of heart disease and stroke, cancers of the prostate, stomach, lungs and breast, and osteoporosis, and protects LDL cholesterol from oxidation, which prevents heart disease.

- Lycopene is non-toxic and can be consumed in large amounts, although eating too much can give the skin a temporary red tint known as lycopenodermia. This condition is considered harmless and will go away on its own when lycopene is no longer consumed.
- Some people may have an intolerance to lycopene and symptoms are similar to gastroenteritis, with onset delayed 12-24 hours from ingestion.
- Natural sources of lycopene are: apricots, asparagus, basil, bell peppers (red), chilli peppers (red), citrus fruits, grapefruit (pink), guava, lettuce (romaine), papaya, parsley, persimmons, red cabbage, rosehips, tomatoes, and watermelon.

*Highest sources of carotenoids (in micrograms (µg) per 100 grams)*

- Chilli powder, paprika 26162 µg
- Sun-dried chilli peppers 14844 µg
- Sweet potatoes 11509 µg
- Kale 8823 µg
- Carrots 8332 µg
- Pumpkin 6940 µg
- Romaine lettuce 5226 µg
- Parsley 5054 µg

- Marjoram 4806 µg
- Sage 4806 µg
- Butternut squash 4570 µg
- Cress 4150 µg
- Coriander 3930 µg
- Basil 3142 µg
- Broccoli 2720 µg
- Chives 2612 µg
- Watercress 1914 µg
- Leeks 1000 µg
- Passion fruit 743 µg
- Courgettes 670 µg
- Mango 640 µg
- Asparagus 604 µg

**NOTE**: Eat all foods rich in carotenoids with fatty foods like avocado, nuts, oily fish, seeds and virgin cold-pressed coconut, olive, rapeseed, rice bran or other plant oils to enable absorption because carotenoids are fat-soluble, meaning they can only be absorbed into the body along with fats. Excess consumption of carotenoids can cause a yellow/orange colour to the skin which is unattractive but harmless.

## Chalcones (yellow)

Chalcones are often responsible for the yellow pigment of many types of flowers, such as daisies and sunflowers, and in plant foods such as: apples, ashitaba, astragalus, beans, cinnamon, citrus fruit (skins), cloves, green tea, hops, liquorice root, peas, potatoes, sunflower seeds and tomato skins.

- They are a class of flavonoid compounds which are potent antioxidants, protecting cells from free-radical damage, which is associated with accelerating the ageing process and with many disorders, including cancer, as well as degenerative diseases. They also suppress the excessive secretion of gastric juice in the stomach, which is often caused by stress and can lead to stomach ulcers.

- In addition, chalcones help to strengthen the immune system, regulate blood pressure and cholesterol and exhibit antiviral and antibacterial activities. They have also been found to stimulate the production of nerve growth factor (NGF), which is synthesised in minute amounts in the body and is essential for the development and survival of certain neurons (nerve cells) in the peripheral and central nervous system. NGF is believed to have the potential to alleviate Alzheimer's disease and peripheral neuropathy (a common neurological disorder resulting from damage to the peripheral nerves, which originate from the spinal cord). In an animal study conducted by the Biomedical Group, in Takara, Japan, there was a 20 per cent increase in NGF concentration after consuming ashitaba leaves for just four days.

## Chlorophyll (green)

Chlorophyll is the green pigment present in plants that is responsible for collecting and storing energy from the sun. It is a molecule that absorbs sunlight and uses its energy to synthesise carbohydrates from carbon dioxide and water in a process known as photosynthesis. Because the chlorophyll molecule is almost identical to the haemoglobin molecule in red blood cells it is often referred to as 'nature's blood'.

- One of its many beneficial properties is its ability to stimulate the production of red blood cells, which carry oxygen to the body's tissues.
- It is also an excellent agent for cleansing the blood, bowels and liver and it promotes the growth of beneficial intestinal bacteria.
- It can also bind with heavy metals and remove them from the body and strengthens immunity. It also has antioxidant and anti-inflammatory properties, alkalises the blood, helps fight off diseases and protects against cancer.

It is for these reasons that it is advisable to consume at least one green leafy vegetable every day.

### Curcumin (yellow)

Turmeric is the bright yellow of the spice rainbow and a powerful medicine that has long been used in the Chinese and Indian systems of medicine as an anti-inflammatory agent to treat a wide variety of conditions, including bacterial infections, bloody urine, flatulence, haemorrhage, jaundice, menstrual difficulties, toothache, bruises, chest pain and colic. It can also provide an inexpensive, well-tolerated and effective treatment for inflammatory bowel diseases such as Crohn's, as well as other conditions such as liver disorders, neurological disorders, peripheral neuropathy and ulcerative colitis.

- Curcumin, the major constituent of turmeric that gives the spice its yellow colour, can correct the most common expression of the genetic defect that is responsible for cystic fibrosis.
- The frequent consumption of turmeric leads to a reduced risk of developing breast, colon, lung and prostate cancers. Even when breast cancer is already present, curcumin can help slow the spread of breast cancer cells to the lungs.
- Curcumin exerts very powerful antioxidant effects and can neutralise free radicals. This is important in many diseases, such as arthritis, where free radicals are responsible for the painful inflammation and eventual damage to the joints. Curcumin's combination of antioxidant and anti-inflammatory effects explains why many people with joint disease find relief when they consume it regularly.
- Turmeric has also been scientifically proven to be more effective at treating depression than many anti-depressant drugs.
- Treatment of brain cells, called astrocytes, with curcumin has been found to increase the expression of glutathione and protect neurons exposed to oxidative stress.
- Increasing turmeric in the diet can increase the levels of the amino acid glutathione in the body which can be beneficial for a huge range of diseases and disorders as it is present in every cell of the body and has an important antioxidant role.

- Prostate cancer is a rare occurrence among men in India, whose low risk is attributed to a diet rich in brassica family vegetables (cauliflower, cabbage, broccoli, Brussels sprouts, kale, kohlrabi and turnips) and the spice, turmeric. Both phenethyl isothiocyanate and curcumin greatly retard the growth of human prostate cancer cells. The combination of cruciferous vegetables and curcumin could be an effective therapy not only to prevent prostate cancer, but to inhibit the spread of established prostate cancers.
- Turmeric is also beneficial for measles.

## Flavins (pale-yellow and green fluorescent)

Flavins are a class of pale-yellow and green fluorescent, water-soluble biochromes widely distributed in small quantities in plant and animal tissues. The most prevalent member of the class is **riboflavin (vitamin B2)**. Flavins are synthesised by bacteria, yeasts and green plants; riboflavin is not manufactured by animals, which therefore are dependent upon plant sources.

- Riboflavin is a component of an enzyme capable of combining with molecular oxygen; the product, which is yellow, releases the oxygen in the cell with simultaneous loss of colour. When supplements containing vitamin B2 are consumed the excess, that is not absorbed, can often be seen as florescent yellow in the urine.
- Vitamin B2 is required by the body to use oxygen and for

the metabolism of amino acids, fatty acids, carbohydrates and protein. It is further needed to activate vitamin B6 (pyridoxine) and vitamin B9 (folic acid), helps to create vitamin B3 (niacin) and assists the adrenal gland. It is also used for red blood cell formation, antibody production, cell respiration and growth. It eases watery eye fatigue and can be helpful in the prevention and treatment of cataracts.

- Vitamin B2 is also required for the health of the mucous membranes in the digestive tract and helps with the absorption of iron and vitamin B6. Although it is needed for periods of rapid growth, it is also required when protein intake is high and is most beneficial to the skin, hair and nails.
- Vitamin B2 helps reduce homocysteine levels in the body thereby reducing the risk of strokes, heart attacks and deaths from heart disease. It also helps reduce the frequency of migraine headaches.
- Vitamin B2 is manufactured industrially using yeast or other fermenting organisms, used as a yellow colouring and as vitamin fortification, but is difficult to incorporate into most foods due to poor solubility and instability upon exposure to light.
- Low levels of vitamin B2 may manifest as cracks and sores at the corners of the mouth, eye disorders, inflammation of the mouth and tongue, skin lesions, dermatitis, dizziness, hair loss, insomnia, light sensitivity, poor digestion, retarded

growth and slow mental responses. Burning feet can also be a sign of a shortage and it can also cause a lack of red blood cells.

*Highest sources of vitamin B2 (in milligrams per 100 grams)*
- Yeast extract 17.5 mg
- Baker's yeast 4 mg
- Parsley 2.38 mg
- Almonds 1.10 mg
- Soya beans 0.76 mg
- Wheat bran 0.58 mg
- Sun-dried tomatoes 0.28 mg
- Spinach 0.21 mg
- Peas 0.12 mg

# How to consume a wide selection of colours

Only small traces of many nutrients are required and such a wide selection of colours can be difficult to consume all in one day due to the bulk of the foods. Often supermarkets sell fruit and vegetables in multipacks meaning much gets wasted and more than enough of one colour is consumed at once at the expense of the others. The best practice is to visit local greengrocers or farmers' markets where they sell their produce by weight or singly and buy one or two of each of the six colours every couple of days depending on the size of the household.

(**Note**: It is difficult for small greengrocers to sell organic foods due to higher costs and they cannot compete with the supermarkets who buy massive amounts in bulk. However, the more people who shop at independent greengrocers instead, and demand organic produce, the quicker we will all be able to enjoy healthier foods and more diversity of colourful fruits and vegetables at lower prices. This will then have the added benefits of improving the overall health of everyone and helping organic farmers and small businesses, such as greengrocers, to thrive.)

### *Making teas*

A good way to consume the colourful nutrients of fruits, herbs, seeds, spices and vegetables, without the bulk, is to make teas with them. Simply pour hot (but not quite boiling) water over them (seeds and spices can be ground into the tea) and allow to steep for 20 minutes, then strain and sip the juice. Try experimenting and making unusual teas by mixing different herbs and spices. Drink three cups a day gently reheated or cold with ice. For tougher stems and roots of vegetables, simply simmer them gently for 15 minutes, then strain and consume as above.

**Note**: Adding a teaspoon of pure honey, the freshly squeezed juices of citrus fruits and a pinch of black pepper can provide further powerful health benefits as well as taste, and including the zest of citrus fruits and two or three cloves will provide additional benefits.

## *Juicing fruit and vegetables*

To make it easier to consume a wider selection of foods, and hence a wider range of nutrients without the bulk, purchase a powerful juicer. The best to use, to get the most nutrients from fruit and vegetables, are the slow juicers of at least 900 watts. In case of incomplete extraction of juices, their effective health benefits are greatly reduced due to the absence of the enzymes, minerals and vitamins which are left behind in fibre and the pulp.

Raw juices have many beneficial effects on our health but should not replace the consumption of whole fruits and vegetables as these provide the vital fibre needed for proper digestion and the correct functioning of the excretory system. The favourable effect of raw juices in the treatment of disease is attributed to the following facts:

- Raw juices of fruits and vegetables are extremely rich in vitamins, minerals, trace elements, enzymes and natural sugars.
- They exercise beneficial effects in normalising all the body's functions.
- They supply needed elements for the body's own healing activity and cell regeneration, thereby speeding recovery and repair.

- The juices extracted from raw fruits and vegetables require minimal digestion and almost all their vital nutrients are absorbed directly into the bloodstream.
- Raw juices are extremely rich in alkaline elements. This is highly beneficial in normalising acid-alkaline balance in the blood and tissues as over-acidity is a known cause of many diseases.
- There are high amounts of easily absorbed organic minerals in raw juices, especially calcium, potassium and silicon, that help in restoring biochemical and mineral balance in the tissues and cells, thereby preventing premature ageing of cells and disease.
- Raw juices contain certain natural medicines, vegetal hormones and antibiotics. For instance, string beans are said to contain an insulin-like substance. Certain hormones needed by the pancreas to produce insulin are present in cucumber and onion juices. Fresh juices of garlic, onions, radish and tomatoes contain antibiotic substances.

## Juices for common ailments

Some common ailments and the fruits and vegetable juices found beneficial in their treatment include:

- **Acidity:** apple, avocado, banana, carrot, grape, pear, mosambi, orange and spinach.
- **Acne:** carrot, cucumber, grape, pear, plum, potato, radish, spinach and tomato.

- **Allergies:** apricot, beetroot, carrot, ginger, grape and spinach.
- **Arteriosclerosis:** apple, beetroot, blueberries, carrot, celery, grapefruit, ginger, grapes (black or red), pineapple, lemon, lettuce, pomegranate, spinach and watercress.
- **Anaemia:** apricot, banana, beetroot, carrot, celery, strawberry, spinach and watercress.
- **Arthritis:** apple (sour), avocado, beetroot, carrot, cherries (sour), cucumber, grapefruit, lemon, lettuce, papaya, pineapple, spinach and watercress.
- **Asthma:** apple, apricot, carrot, celery, lemon, pineapple, peach, radish and strawberry.
- **Bladder and kidney disorders:** apple, apricot, blueberries, carrot, celery, cranberries, cucumber, grapes, lemon and watercress.
- **Bronchitis and respiratory disorders:** apple, apricot, carrot, kiwi fruit, lemon, onion, pineapple, peach, strawberry, spinach and tomato.
- **Colds:** blackberries, carrot, celery, grapefruit, lemon, lime, kiwifruit, onion, orange, pineapple, radish, spinach, tangerine and watercress.
- **Colitis:** apple, apricot, pear, peach, pineapple, papaya, carrot, beet, cucumber and spinach.
- **Constipation:** apple, banana, beetroot, carrot, ginger, grapes, lemon, pear, plums, spinach and watercress.
- **Cystitis:** apple, apricot, blueberries, carrot, celery,

cranberries, cucumber, grapes, lemon and watercress.

- **Diabetes:** broccoli, cabbage, carrot, celery, citrus fruits, guava, lettuce, radish, spinach and watercress.
- **Diarrhoea:** avocado, carrot, celery, lemon, papaya and pineapple.
- **Digestive disorders:** apple, apricot, avocado, banana, carrot, ginger, grapes, pear, mosambi, orange and spinach.
- **Eczema:** avocado, beetroot, blueberries, carrot, cucumber, grapes (black or red), spinach and watercress.
- **Epilepsy:** carrot, celery, coriander, grape (red or black), spinach and watercress.
- **Eye disorders:** apricot, avocado, bilberries, blackberries, blueberries, carrot, celery, cranberries, raspberries, spinach, strawberries, tomato and watercress.
- **Gout:** beetroot, carrot, celery, cherries (sour), cucumber, pineapple, tomato and watercress.
- **Halitosis:** apple, carrot, celery, grapefruit, lemon, pineapple, spinach and tomato.
- **Haemorrhoids:** carrot, lemon, orange, papaya, pineapple, spinach, turnip and watercress.
- **Headache and migraine:** avocado, carrot, cherries (sour), coriander, grapes, lemon, lettuce, papaya, pineapple, spinach and watercress.
- **Heart disease:** apple, banana, beetroot, carrot, cucumber, ginger, grapes (black or red), lemon, pomegranate, spinach and watercress.

- **High blood pressure:** banana, beetroot, carrot, cucumber, ginger, grapes, orange and watercress.
- **Influenza:** apricot, blackberries, carrot, ginger, grapefruit, lemon, onion, orange, pineapple, radish, spinach and watercress.
- **Insomnia:** apple, banana, carrot, celery, cherries (sour), grapes, lemon, lettuce and tomato.
- **Jaundice and liver disorders:** beetroot, carrot, cranberry, cucumber, ginger, grapes, lemon, papaya, pear, radish, spinach and tomato.
- **Menopausal symptoms:** apricot, banana, beetroot, carrot, celery, grape (black or red), lemon, papaya, plum, spinach, strawberry, tomato and watercress.
- **Menstrual disorders:** beetroot, cherries (sour), ginger, grapes, lettuce, plums, spinach, turnips and watercress.
- **Neuritis:** apple, avocado, beetroot, blueberries, carrot, orange, papaya, pineapple, radish and watercress.
- **Obesity:** apple, beetroot, cabbage, carrot, celery, grapefruit, lemon, lettuce, orange, pineapple, papaya, radish, spinach, tangerine, tomato and watercress.
- **Pleurisy:** apple, carrot, cranberry, grapes, lemon, lime, onion, orange, papaya, pineapple, radish, spinach, strawberry, tangerine and tomato.
- **Pneumonia:** apple, avocado, kiwifruit, orange, mosambi, apple, papaya, pineapple, garlic, radish, grapes, carrots, tangerine and tomatoes.

- **Prostate problems:** apple, apricot, asparagus, blueberries, carrot, celery, cranberry, cucumber, lettuce, spinach, tomatoes and watercress.
- **Psoriasis:** apple, apricot, beetroot, carrot, cucumber, grapes, lemon and watercress.
- **Rheumatism:** beetroot, carrot, cherries (sour), cucumber, grapefruit, grapes, lemon, orange, papaya, pineapple, spinach, tomato and watercress.
- **Sinus trouble:** apricot, carrot, ginger, lemon, onion, radish and tomato.
- **Sore throat:** apricot, carrot, ginger, grapes, lemon, pineapple, plums and tomato.
- **Stomach ulcers:** apricot, avocado, cabbage, carrot and grapes.
- **Tonsillitis:** apricot, carrot, lemon, ginger, grapefruit, orange, pineapple, radish, spinach and watercress.
- **Varicose veins:** beetroot, carrot, ginger, grapes, orange, plum, radish, tomato, turnips and watercress.

**NOTE:** Avoid grapefruit if taking any medications. Ginger may increase the risk of bleeding if taking any blood thinning medications.

## Types of juices

Fruit and vegetable juices may be divided into six main types:

1. Juices from sweet fruits such as prunes, raisins and grapes.
2. Juices from sub-acid fruits like apples, plums, pears,

peaches, papaya, apricots and cherries.

3. Juices from acid fruits like oranges, tangerines, lemons, grapefruit, strawberries and pineapples.
4. Juices from vegetable fruits, namely tomatoes and cucumber.
5. Juices from green leafy vegetables like cabbage, celery, lettuce, spinach, parsley and watercress.
6. Juices from root vegetables like beetroot, carrot, onion, potato and radish.

Fruit juices are said to stimulate the body's eliminative processes. Vegetable juices, on the other hand, soothe the jaded nerves and work in a much milder manner to carry away toxic matter. Owing to their differing actions, fruit and vegetable juices should not be used at the same time or mixed together. It is desirable to use juices individually. Ideally not more than three juices should be used in any one mixture.

## Rules for making juices

- Juices from sweet fruits may be combined with juices of sub-acid fruits, but not with those of acid fruits, vegetable fruits or vegetables.
- Juices from sub-acid fruits may be combined with juices of sweet fruits, or acid fruits, but not with other juices.
- Juices from acid fruits may be combined with those of sub-acid fruits or vegetable fruits, but not with other juices.

- Juices from vegetable fruits may be combined with those of acid fruits or of green leafy vegetables, but not with other juices.
- Juices from green leafy vegetables may be combined with those of vegetable fruits or of the root vegetable, but not with other juices.
- Juices from root vegetables may be combined with those of green leafy vegetables, but not with other juices.

A correct selection of juices is essential in addressing a particular ailment. For instance, juices of carrot, cucumber, cabbage and other vegetables are very valuable in asthma, arthritis and skin disease, but juices of orange and mosambi aggravate the symptoms by increasing the amount of mucus.

**Note:** To make juicing tastier many beneficial herbs, spices and condiments may be added according to taste. All are very helpful in cleansing the system and fighting bacteria and cancer. Particularly: organic apple cider vinegar, pure organic honey, turmeric, black pepper, cayenne pepper, cumin, cinnamon, ginger, basil, oregano, thyme, coriander, fennel, parsley, dill, low-fat live yoghurt and coconut milk.

### Raw juicing methods

- When on a raw-juice regime, the recommended juice should be drunk every three hours. One can thus take juices five to six times a day.

- A warm glass of water mixed with lemon juice, one teaspoon of honey, a dash of vinegar plus a small pinch of cayenne pepper may be taken first thing in the morning on rising to help the toxin cleanse.
- Thereafter, the recommended juice may be taken at three-hourly intervals. The quantity of juice on each occasion may be 250 ml on the first day.
- This quantity may be increased by 50 ml each succeeding day until one takes 600 ml on each occasion.
- The juice diet can be continued for 30 to 40 days without any ill effects. The patient should take adequate rest during the raw-juice therapy.
- Raw juices act as a cleansing agent and start eliminating toxins matter from the system immediately. This often results in symptoms such as pain in the abdomen, diarrhoea, loss of weight, headache, fever, weakness, sleeplessness and bad breath. These reactions, which are part of the cleansing process, should not be suppressed with drugs. They will cease when the body has been able to expel all toxins.
- After the raw-juice therapy, the return to a normal balanced diet should be gradual and in stages. In the beginning, two juice meals may be replaced by milk (unless there is an intolerance) and fruits. Then gradually juice meals may be substituted by a balanced diet.
- Make sure all vegetables and fruits are washed thoroughly

and drip dried before juicing and, where possible, buy organic for the greatest benefit.

- Generally speaking, a masticating juicer is the best type to use for juicing green vegetables, cereal grasses, sprouted shoots such as alfalfa sprouts, immature sunflower and buckwheat plants. This kind of juicer moves at low speed and squeezes the material, while preserving healthy and beneficial qualities of the produce.

- To maximize nutritious benefits, use the freshest ingredients available, ideally picked immediately before juicing, and drink immediately.

- Juicing shouldn't be a substitute for eating whole fruits and vegetables. There are other essentials such as fibre, which are lost in juicing. However, if having a juice fast, detoxifying, or recovering from illness, juicing is a superb way of getting concentrated nutrients in an easily assimilated form.

- Dark-green leafy vegetable juices are highly beneficial because of their chlorophyll and high antioxidant content; this means they are more effective at eliminating toxic waste compounds from the body.

- Adding herbs like basil, coriander and parsley leaves to the juices will add flavour as well as further detoxifying benefits.

- Juicing is also a great way to break down the often false barriers between culinary and medicinal herbs, by bringing highly nutritional herbs like ashitaba, drumstick leaves, seaweed and dandelion leaves into the everyday diet.

- Other types of greens that can be added sparingly (because they are very bitter) include kale, collard greens and mustard greens.

## Nature Cures healthy juicing recipes

Imagination can be used to make blends that suit the palate and ailment, but below are some recipes to get started with. Plain yoghurt with live cultures can be added to juices after they have been made to make a creamy smoothie. Apple cider vinegar has amazing medicinal properties and can also be added to juices, as can honey if the juice is too sour. Adding unrefined sea salt and black pepper can provide more nutrients and minerals as well as taste.

- Skins can be left on most vegetables (except hard rinds on pumpkins etc) but remove any large stones such as avocado, apricot, peach etc.
- Chopping vegetables, fruits and herbs can help them pass through the juicer more effectively.
- Juice the ingredients in the order they are listed. Harder vegetables, like celery and cucumber, help flush the fibres of the leafy greens through the juicer. Stir spices and liquids, such as coconut juice or apple cider vinegar, into the juice afterwards.
- Wash the juicer parts immediately to stop the pulp drying hard.

## ALOE GREEN HIGH-NUTRITION JUICE

Aloe boosts the immune system, reduces inflammation, improves skin health, stabilises blood sugar levels in diabetics, lowers LDL cholesterol and triglycerides and amplifies the antioxidant effects of vitamins. This is also a great juice for the relief of heartburn.

- Three inches of aloe vera leaf or 4 oz of aloe vera juice (added after juicing the other ingredients)
- Half an inch of ginger
- One fennel bulb
- Two kale leaves
- Two carrots
- One apple
- One lemon
- Five stalks of celery.

## ANTI-CANCER, ANTIOXIDANT AND PURIFYING JUICE

The mono-unsaturated fat in avocado helps absorption of the fat-soluble and cancer-fighting carotenoid lycopene in tomatoes, making it four times as effective. Other sources of lycopene are apricots, asparagus, basil, chilli peppers, grapefruit (pink), guava, papaya, parsley, persimmons, red cabbage, rosehips and watermelon.

- Four medium tomatoes (or 10 baby tomatoes)
- One red pepper (de-seeded)
- One avocado pear
- Half a lemon
- Small handful of fresh basil and/or parsley leaves

- One stick of celery
- Pinch of chilli pepper powder
- Black pepper

## ANTI-INFLAMMATORY PAIN RELIEVER
- Handful of sour cherries
- Five to eight basil leaves
- One papaya
- Half an inch of ginger
- Quarter of a pineapple
- One tablespoon of ground hemp or chia seeds stirred in afterwards
- One coconut (remove flesh from shell and juice then stir in the coconut juice).

## BLADDER, KIDNEY AND LIVER CLEANSER
To help burn fat, detoxify and clean the urinary system.
- One dandelion root
- A small handful of basil
- One beetroot + green top
- One apple
- Two carrots
- One stalk of celery.

## BRAIN, COLON, HEART AND PROSTATE PROTECTOR
Kale, a rich source of carotene, indoles, vitamins A, C, K and the B

vitamins, plus calcium and iron, together with the other ingredients can prevent colon, heart, neurological and prostate disorders.

- Three leaves of kale
- One handful of watercress
- One handful of coriander leaves
- One avocado (stone removed)
- One apple
- One red bell pepper
- Three carrots.

**CHOLESTEROL-LOWERING JUICE**
- Half an inch of ginger
- One avocado (stone removed)
- One pomegranate (cut in half and scoop insides into the juicer)
- One apple
- Five radishes
- Three carrots.

## Precautions when juicing

Certain precautions are necessary in adopting a diet of raw juices:

1. All juices should be made fresh immediately before drinking. Canned and frozen juices should not be used.
2. Only washed, fresh and ripe fruits and vegetables, preferably organically grown, should be used for extraction of juices.
3. Only as much juice as needed for immediate consumption

should be extracted. Raw juices oxidise rapidly and lose their medicinal value in storage, even under refrigeration.

4. The quality of the juices has a distinct bearing on the results obtained. In case of incomplete extraction of juices, their effective power is proportionately reduced due to the absence of the vitamins and enzymes which are left behind in fibre and the pulp. A slow juicer of at least 900 watts is required to obtain the health benefits mentioned in this pocketbook.

5. If juices are too sweet they should be diluted in water on a 50:50 basis, or mixed with other less sweet juices. This is especially important in some specific conditions, such as diabetes, hypoglycaemia, arthritis and high blood pressure.

## *What colourful foods to avoid and when*

As with everything in life, moderation is the secret to good health, contentment and wellbeing. Even the excessive consumption of water can be toxic to the human body as it affects the concentration of minerals in the blood and cells. Also, in some cases certain foods, even the healthiest and richest in nutrients, can cause complications. For instance, grapefruit should be avoided if taking certain medications as it can react and either weaken or strengthen their effect, especially those that lower cholesterol and blood pressure. The following is a guide to other foods and circumstances where they should be avoided.

- Allspice if suffering from stomach ulcers, ulcerative colitis or diverticulitis.

- Almonds, cabbage and kale, plums and prunes if suffering from gout, bladder stones, gallstones or kidney stones, joint problems, osteoporosis or thyroid gland problems.
- Aloe vera, cats claw, dandelion, Echinacea and astragalus if pregnant or breast feeding or have high blood pressure.
- Angelica (dong quai), cumin, ginger, Japanese knotweed, motherwort and turmeric if taking anticoagulants (blood thinning medication), hormone therapies, contraceptive or non-steroidal anti-inflammatory medications, such as aspirin and ibuprofen, or have heart problems and during the first trimester of pregnancy.
- Chinese rhubarb root is not recommended for long-term use and is not suitable for pregnant or breast feeding women, children under 12 years of age, those who suffer from colitis or have an intestinal obstruction or have a history of kidney stones or urinary problems, or if taking anticoagulant (blood thinning) medicine or aspirin.
- Chlorella and spirulina if suffering from a seafood or iodine allergy, a metabolic condition called phenylketonuria (PKU), multiple sclerosis, rheumatoid arthritis or lupus. If pregnant or nursing or have hyperthyroidism, consult a healthcare provider before taking spirulina. It may interfere with medications to suppress the immune system.
- Devil's claw if diabetic or taking blood pressure or blood-thinning medications.
- Ginseng if pregnant or breastfeeding or suffering from

asthma, emphysema, fibrocystic breasts, high blood pressure, clotting problems or cardiac arrhythmia.

- Goji berries if taking medication for diabetes, high blood pressure or anti-coagulants (blood thinners), such as warfarin or aspirin.
- Grapefruit can interact with many types of medications, such as statins or blood pressure medications amongst others, by reducing or increasing their effectiveness.
- Land caltrop can cause miscarriage and must be avoided by pregnant or breastfeeding women or individuals with breast or prostate cancer. Excess consumption of land caltrop can cause sleep disturbances and irregular menstruation and high doses may adversely affect the eyes and liver.
- Linden if suffering from heart disease or are pregnant or breastfeeding or if taking diuretics as it could increase the concentration of lithium in the blood.
- Liquorice root if suffering from high blood pressure, a heart condition, oedema or are taking certain medications such as warfarin or diuretics.
- Marshmallow herb if suffering from diabetes, alcohol dependency or liver disease or if pregnant or breastfeeding.
- Motherwort may be habit forming.
- Nettles if suffering from heart or kidney problems.
- Poke root if pregnant or breastfeeding, and do not give to children.
- Reishi mushrooms if taking anti-hypertensive, blood sugar

lowering or anticoagulant medications or are pregnant.

- Rosemary if pregnant or breastfeeding or suffering from high blood pressure.
- Sage if pregnant or suffering from epilepsy.
- Scutellaria if pregnant or breastfeeding.
- Senega root if hypersensitive to salicylates or aspirin or pregnant.
- Siberian ginseng if suffering from high blood pressure or anxiety.
- Swiss chard if there is an existing and untreated kidney or gallbladder problem.
- Whole nuts and seeds if suffering from diverticulitis (grind to a fine powder first).

Many herbs are powerful and can react with medications, especially astragalus, cats claw, dandelion, and echinacea. Always check before taking at the same time as any drugs.

**NOTE:** Avoid yohimbine and ginseng under any of the following circumstances:

- Allergic hypersensitivity
- Angina pectoris and cardiac disease
- Anxiety
- Asthma
- Cardiac arrhythmia
- Children under 16 years' old
- Clotting problems
- Depression
- Elderly (over 60)

- Emphysema
- Fibrocystic breasts
- Heart disease
- High blood pressure
- Kidney disease
- Liver disease
- Pregnant or breastfeeding
- Prostatitis
- Schizophrenia

## Artificial colours

When 'eating the rainbow' it is essential to be aware of what is natural colour in any food and what has been added. Synthetic food colours are added to foods as a cheap way of making the food look more appetising and pleasing to the eye. Unfortunately, many cause serious side effects and a number have been banned by some countries in the developed world, especially Norway, but are still being used by many others, including the UK and USA.

These artificial food colours confuse the picture, where nature's colour codes are concerned, as they bear no relationship to naturally-occurring pigments and nutrition. Some (see below) have been tested on animals and proven to be carcinogenic, but long-term tests on humans have not yet been carried out. Chemicals used as food dyes have been given the E numbers from E100 to E199 by the European Food Safety Authority. At the time of going to press the following was accurate but approvals or the banning of some food dyes may have changed in some countries since then.

'Natural' food dyes are produced from plants using hexane, acetone and other solvents to break down cell walls in fruit and vegetables and allow for maximum extraction of the colour. Traces of these solvents may remain in the finished colorant, but they do not need to be declared on the product label. These solvents are known as carry-over ingredients. Hexane is a chemical made from crude oil that can cause nerve damage and paralysis of the arms and legs.

Synthetic coal tar dyes are artificial colouring agents made by combining various aromatic hydrocarbons, such as benzene, toluene and xylene, which are obtained from the distillation of bituminous coal. Azo dyes are coal tar dyes whose molecules contain two adjacent nitrogen atoms between carbon atoms. Azo dyes are formed from an azoic diazo component and a coupling component. The first compound, an aniline, gives a diazonium salt upon treatment with nitrous acid and this salt reacts with the coupling component to form a dye. Azo dyes derived from benzidine are carcinogens and exposure to them has been associated with bladder cancer.

Benzene is known to cause cancer, based on evidence from studies in both people and laboratory animals - mainly leukaemia and other cancers of blood cells.

Toluene is a toxic chemical used in nail products and hair dyes. It is added to gasoline and used to produce benzene and as a solvent. Exposure to toluene can result in temporary effects such as headaches, dizziness and cracked skin, as well as more serious effects, such as reproductive damage and respiratory complications.

Xylene is manufactured from petroleum and composed of three isomers (ortho-, meta-, and para-xylene), characterised as a colourless, sweet-smelling and highly flammable liquid. It occurs naturally in petroleum and coal tar. Xylene is used as a solvent in paints and inks and as a cleaning agent.

### Dyes and lakes

Colour additives are produced for use in food as either 'dyes' or 'lakes'.

Dyes dissolve in water, but are not soluble in oil and are manufactured as powders, granules, liquids or other special purpose forms. They can be found in baked goods, beverages, confectionary, dairy products, dry food mixes, pet foods and a variety of other products.

Lakes are made by combining dyes with salts (usually aluminium salts) to make insoluble compounds. Lakes are not oil-soluble, but are oil-dispersible and are more stable than dyes. They are suited to colouring products containing fats and oils or items lacking sufficient moisture to dissolve dyes, such as cake and doughnut mixes, coated pharmaceutical tablets, hard sweets and chewing gums, lipsticks, shampoos, soaps and talcum powder etc.

**Artificial dyes are divided into three categories**

1. Suitable for foods, drugs, and cosmetics
2. Suitable only for drugs and cosmetics
3. Suitable only for cosmetics

Because drugs and cosmetics also get absorbed into the body this guidance is not appropriate and all E numbers should be avoided due to the risk of allergic reactions, adverse neurological effects and cancer.

Unfortunately, bright synthetic colours make food attractive to children and it is these colours that can adversely affect children's health the most. This is at a critical time when a child needs to be healthy and able to learn and develop. The effects of additives could have repercussions on the education and personality of a child for the rest of his or her life.

## Signs that a child is being affected by E-numbers in foods

- Anxiety and/or depression
- Asthma attacks
- Concentration issues
- Hyperactivity
- Irritability
- Oppositional defiance
- Restlessness or difficulty falling asleep

- Rashes
- Temper tantrums.

Avoidance of all E-numbered food additives, by carefully checking ingredient labels, is the best practice.

## *Food colourings in common use*

**E100** Curcumin is a natural yellow/orange food colouring derived from the turmeric (*Curcuma longa*) rhizome, but excessive consumption can cause hives, migraines, nausea, rashes and an increased risk of bleeding in anyone taking anticoagulants ('blood thinners') or women who are pregnant.

*Products that may contain E100*
- Biscuits
- Butter
- Carbonated drinks
- Cheese
- Fish fingers
- Margarine

**E102** Tartrazine (Yellow #5) is a bright yellow/orange azo dye that can cause asthma, anxiety, behavioural issues, blurred vision, chromosomal damage to the foetus, depression, hyperactivity, migraines, purple patches and rashes on the skin and thyroid cancer. E102 appears to cause the most allergic reactions of all the azo dyes, particularly in individuals who are asthmatic or have an aspirin intolerance. It is often used with E133 (Brilliant Blue FCF, see page 71) to produce various green shades for different products, such as tinned processed peas. It is very commonly used in the UK and other countries despite being banned by Austria and Norway.

*Products that may contain E102*
- Alcoholic mixers
- Baked goods
- Beer
- Breakfast cereals
- Butter and margarine
- Cake mixes and instant desserts
- Cheeses (orange coloured)
- Chewing gum
- Chicken broth (cubed or powered)
- Confectionary and sweets
- Cosmetics, body washes, conditioners, moisturisers, shampoos, shaving creams.
- Crackers and crisps
- Custard powder
- Fizzy drinks
- Frosting
- Fruit cordials and squashes
- Glycerine, lemon and honey products
- Ice cream and ice lollies

- Jam
- Jelly
- Macaroni cheese
- Marmalade
- Marzipan
- Medicinal capsule shells
- Milk (flavoured)
- Mustard
- Pancake mix
- Pasta
- Pet foods
- Pickles
- Ready meals with cheese flavourings
- Vitamin supplements (chewable)
- Tinned processed peas
- Yoghurt.

**E103** Alkanet (Alkannin) is a yellow/orange/burgundy colour that is obtained from the extracts of plants from the borage family, (*Alkanna tinctorial*, found in the south of France). It has been shown to increase hyperactivity in affected children, adversely affect those who are sensitive to aspirin and cause allergic reactions such as asthma and hives (nettle-type rashes). It is not approved for use in foods in Europe and is unlisted in the USA but is still used in Australia, Canada and New Zealand.

*Products that may contain E104*

- Cosmetics
- Indian food such as Rogan josh
- Wine
- Wine bottle corks to make wines look aged.

**E104** Quinoline yellow (FD&C Yellow No.10) is a synthetic coal tar dye (disodium salt of disulphonic acid) varying in colour between a dull yellow and greenish-yellow. It has been shown to cause cancer, eye damage and blindness, hyperactivity (ADHD) in children and tumours and, when used in cosmetics, it can cause dermatitis. It is banned in Australia, Japan, Norway and the USA but commonly used in the UK.

*Products that may contain E104*

- Colognes
- Hair products
- Lipsticks
- Medications
- Scotch eggs
- Smoked haddock.

**E105** Fast Yellow AB, (Fast Yellow, Acid Yellow, C.I. 13015, C.I. 14270 or Food Yellow 2) is banned in Europe and the USA due to its harmful toxic properties.

**E107** Yellow 2G (Acid yellow 17, CI Food yellow #5) is an azo coal tar dye used in soft drinks and industrially in printing inks. It was banned in Australia (1992) and is now banned in Austria, Belgium, Denmark, France, Germany, Japan, Norway, Sweden, Switzerland and the USA. It can cause asthma, rashes and hyperactivity and people sensitive to aspirin and asthma sufferers should avoid it.

**E110** Sunset Yellow FCF (Orange Yellow S, Yellow #6) has been known to cause abdominal pain, allergic reactions, bronchial constriction, chromosomal damage, distaste for food, eye damage and blindness, hyperactivity, indigestion and gastric upset, kidney tumours, nasal congestion, nausea and vomiting, rhinitis (runny nose), swelling of the blood vessels and urticaria (hives). It is potentially dangerous to asthmatics and is known to upset some of the digestive enzymes. It has also been linked to growth retardation and severe weight loss in animal tests and increased incidence of tumours in animals. It is banned in Finland, Norway and the UK.

*Products that may contain E110*
- Baked goods
- Cakes
- Carbonated drinks
- Cheese
- Cereals

- Confectionary and sweets
- Dessert mixes
- Ice cream and ice lollies
- Macaroni cheese
- Medications, supplements and cough syrups
- Soft drinks and squashes
- Sauces
- Snacks
- Soups
- Jams and jellies
- Tinned fish
- Yoghurt.

**E120** Cochineal (Carminic acid, Carmines, Red #4) is a natural red colour obtained by crushing the female *Dactilopius coccus*, a cactus-dwelling insect indigenous to Central America. The dye is expensive due to the sheer quantity of shells required to produce a small amount. Alcoholic drinks may contain the water-soluble form (ammonium carmine), but the insoluble calcium carmine is found in many more products. Other non-food uses include as an anti-neoplastic (anti-cancer) agent. It can cause hyperactivity in children and urticaria (hives) and should be avoided by asthmatics, rhinitis sufferers and anyone sensitive to aspirin. It can cause an anaphylactic-shock reaction in some individuals and is banned in the USA.

*Products that may contain E120*

- Alcoholic beverages
- Cakes
- Chewing gum
- Confectionary and sweets
- Dyed cheeses
- Fizzy drinks
- Green vegetables
- Icings
- Parsley sauce
- Pie fillings
- Puddings
- Sauces
- Soups.

**E121** Citrus red (Red #2) is a food dye which is extracted from several species of lichen, also known as orchella weeds. E121 produces an orange to yellow colour, and can also be a dark red powder and has been shown to cause bladder tumours in animal studies. It is used in many products in Europe but is only permitted to colour orange skins in the USA.

*Products that may contain E121*

- Confectionary
- Gravy granules
- Mint sauce

- Ice cream
- Desserts
- Tinned peas

**E122** Azorubine (Carmoisine) is a synthetic red food dye from the azo dye group. Azorubine is commonly used in the UK. A study commissioned by the UK's Food Standards Agency found that when used in a mixture of preservatives, increased levels of hyperactivity in children were observed. The process of making synthetic dyes is via treatment of sulphuric acid or nitric acid that is often contaminated by arsenic or other heavy metals, which are toxic. Consuming foods that contain excessive carmoisine may cause allergic skin reactions and can lead to cancer. It can also adversely affect those that are sensitive to aspirin. It is banned in Austria, Japan, Norway, Sweden and the United States.

*Products that may contain E122*
- Blancmange
- Breadcrumbs
- Cheesecake mixes
- Desserts
- Drinks (red coloured)
- Jams and preserves
- Jellies
- Marzipan
- Red mouthwashes

- Swiss roll
- Yoghurts.

**E123** Amaranth should not to be confused with 'palatable amaranth', a small, highly nutritious, protein-rich seed often used as an alternative to grains. E123 Amaranth is a purple-red synthetic coal tar or azo dye used for colouring in food. It is introduced as either a powder, in granules or as aluminium lakes. It is added to processed foods and drinks to make them appear more appetising. Because amaranth is an azo dye, it has been proven to provoke asthma, eczema and hyperactivity as well as allergic reactions, similar to nettle rash, among asthmatics and individuals who are sensitive to aspirin. The FDA in the United States has banned E123 amaranth and it is also banned in Austria, Japan, Norway, Russia and Sweden. Except for use in caviar, this synthetic colourant is also restricted in France and Italy.

*Products that may contain E123*
- Alcoholic beverages
- Blackcurrant and red drinks
- Cake mixes and desserts
- Caviar
- Gravy granules
- Ice cream
- Jams and preserves
- Jelly

- Meat patties
- Pie fillings
- Prawns
- Soups
- Tinned fruit
- Trifles.

**E124** Ponceau 4R (Cochineal Red A) is a red synthetic azo dye that can increase hyperactivity in affected children; asthmatics sometimes react badly to it. It can also adversely affect those that are sensitive to aspirin and has been shown to be a carcinogen in animals. It is estimated that one in 10,000 people are allergic to E124. It is banned in Canada, Norway and the USA (in 1976 for being a cancer-causing agent) and restricted in Sweden.

*Products that may contain E124*
- Dessert mixes
- Salami
- Soups
- Tinned fruit
- Toppings.

**E127** Erythrosine (Red #3) is a cherry-pink/red synthetic dye derived from coal tar, that has been shown to cause sensitivity to light and has been associated with learning difficulties. As the erythrosine molecule contains iodide, which may be released as the molecule degrades, it can also increase thyroid hormone levels, leading to hyperthyroidism, and was shown to cause thyroid cancer in rats in a study in 1990. (Food processing at temperatures above 200°C can cause this degradation/iodide release.) It may increase hyperactivity in affected children, asthmatics sometimes react badly to it and it can adversely affect those that are sensitive to aspirin. It is also implicated in photo-toxicity (sensitivity to light).

It is used as a biological stain and serves as an adsorption and fluorescent indicator, a dental plaque-disclosing agent and a radiopaque medium. It is also used to kill maggots (fly larvae) and is toxic to some strains of yeast cells.

Erythrosine is banned in Norway and was banned in the USA in January 1990, but not recalled by the United States FDA.

*Products that may contain E127*
- Bakery products
- Biscuits
- Cakes
- Cherry, rhubarb and strawberry packet desserts
- Chocolate
- Cocktail, glacé and tinned cherries
- Confectionery and sweets
- Custard
- Snack foods
- Dressed crab

- Garlic sausage
- Luncheon meat
- Spreads and pâté
- Printing inks
- Salmon spread
- Scotch eggs
- Stuffed olives
- Tinned fruit
- Trifles.

**E128** Red 2G is a synthetic azo dye which is used particularly in meat products. There is evidence that it can be converted to the substance aniline in the gut; laboratory tests have shown that aniline causes anaemia in rats, as it affects haemoglobin in red blood cells. It may also cause rashes. E128 should be avoided by hyperactive children, asthmatics and people who are sensitive to aspirin and is thought to cause damage to genes and therefore be carcinogenic when added to foods. It is banned in Australia, Austria, Belgium, Canada, Denmark, Germany, Japan, New Zealand, Switzerland, the USA and many other places except the UK.

*Products that may contain E128*

- Jams
- Processed meats and sausages
- Soft drinks.

**E129** Allura Red AC (Red #40) is an orange/red synthetic azo dye introduced in the early 1980s to replace E123 Amaranth in the USA where E123 is prohibited. It is believed to produce a slightly less severe reaction in asthmatics and individuals who are intolerant of aspirin; however, allura red has also been linked to cancer of the immune system in laboratory animals and has been banned in Austria, Belgium, Denmark, France, Germany, Norway, Sweden and Switzerland. Individuals with skin sensitivities are advised to avoid E129.

*Products that may contain E129*
- Biscuits
- Cake mixes
- Cherry pie mixes
- Condiments
- Confectionary and sweets
- Cosmetics
- Dairy products
- Drugs
- Fruit cocktails
- Fruit flavoured fillings
- Gelatine
- Ice cream
- Maraschino cherries
- Puddings.

**E131** Patent Blue V is a synthetic blue/violet dye derived from coal tar and used only moderately in the food industry, for example, in Scotch eggs. It is mainly used as an investigative dye in medical procedures - to colour the lymph vessels and cardiovascular system. It is also used as an acid-base (pH) indicator.

Hypersensitivity reactions have been reported that include itching and nettle-type rash, nausea, low blood pressure and, in rare cases, anaphylactic shock. Asthmatics sometimes react badly and it can adversely affect those who are sensitive to aspirin. Anyone with allergies or intolerances should be cautious. It is banned in Australia, Norway, Japan, New Zealand and the USA.

**E132** Indigotine (Indigo Carmine, Blue #2) is a blue synthetic dye derived from coal tar. The chemical structure of indigo was determined by Prussian chemist JFW Adolf von Baeyer in 1883. As well as being used to colour the food products listed below, it is used in diagnostic medicine as a photometric detector and a biological stain in kidney function tests. It can increase hyperactivity in some children, asthmatics sometimes react badly to it and it can adversely affect those who are sensitive to aspirin; it should be taken with caution by individuals with any kind of allergies or intolerances. It may also cause brain tumours, breathing problems, high blood pressure, nausea and vomiting and rashes and other allergic reactions. It is banned in Norway.

*Products that may contain E132*

- Baked goods
- Biscuits
- Cereals
- Confectionary and sweets
- Ice cream
- Medications (tablets and capsules)
- Milk desserts
- Pet foods
- Sports drinks.

**E133** Brilliant Blue FCF (Blue #1) is a blue synthetic polycyclic aromatic hydrocarbon, triphenylmethane dye usually occurring as an aluminium lake (solution) or ammonium salt. It may increase hyperactivity in affected children and can cause chromosomal damage, bronchial constriction (combined with E127 and E132) and rashes. It was banned in the British Commonwealth 1972-1980 and is now banned in Austria, Belgium, France, Germany, Norway Switzerland and Sweden.

*Products that may contain E133*

- Confectionary and sweets
- Dairy products
- Drinks (soda)
- Inks
- Fabric and wood dye

- Pet foods
- Protein stain
- Sports drinks.

**E142** Green S is a green synthetic dye derived from coal tar. It can cause and worsen asthma and hyperactivity and has caused rashes and cancer in animal tests. It is banned in Canada, Japan, Norway, Sweden and the USA.

*Products that may contain E142*
- Cake mixes
- Mint jelly and sauce
- Packaged breadcrumbs
- Tinned peas

**E150a** Plain caramel
**E150b** Caustic sulphite caramel
**E150c** Ammonia caramel
**E150d** Sulphite ammonia caramel
E150a-d are dark-brown colours made from sucrose in the presence of ammonia, ammonium sulphate, sulphur dioxide or sodium hydroxide. The types of caramel colour available include plain (spirit) caramel (prepared by controlled heat treatment of carbohydrates with or without an acid or base), caustic sulphite caramel (produced by heat treatment of carbohydrates with sulphur-containing compounds), ammonia caramel

(heat treatment in the presence of ammonia) and sulphite ammonia caramel. These should all be avoided as they can cause hyperactivity. Some caramels may also damage genes, slow down growth, cause enlargement of the intestines and kidneys and may destroy B vitamins.

The caramel group of colours are the most widely used, comprising 98 per cent of all colours used. Because these caramels can be derived from malt syrup, milk and wheat products, individuals with allergies or sensitivities to these substances should avoid the 150-colour range of dyes.

*Products that may contain E150a, E150b, E150c and E150d*
- Beer (especially stouts)
- Biscuits
- Brandy
- Bread
- Cakes
- Chocolate
- Confectionary and sweets
- Crisps
- Decorations and coatings
- Dessert mixes
- Doughnuts
- Fillings and toppings
- Fish and shellfish spreads
- Fizzy drinks

- Flour products
- Frozen desserts
- Fruit sauces
- Glucose tablets
- Gravy mixes
- Ice cream
- Jams and preserves
- Milk desserts
- Oyster sauce
- Pancakes
- Pâté
- Pickles
- Sauces and dressings
- Soft drinks (cola etc)
- Soy sauce
- Vinegar
- Whiskey
- Wine
- Vegetable protein and similar meat substitutes.

E151 Brilliant Black BN (Black PN) is a brown/black/violet synthetic azo dye that can be carcinogenic. It can increase hyperactivity in affected children, asthmatics sometimes react badly to it and it can adversely affect those that are sensitive to aspirin. Individuals with any kind of allergies or intolerances should avoid this additive. It may cause urticaria (nettle-type rash) and problems for rhinitis sufferers and is known to interfere with some digestive enzymes. It is banned in Australia, Austria, Belgium, Denmark, France, Germany, Norway, Switzerland, and the USA and greatly restricted in Sweden.

*Products that may contain E151*
- Blackcurrant cake mixes
- Brown sauces
- Confectionary and sweets
- Decorations
- Desserts
- Fish paste
- Flavoured milk drinks
- Fruit jams (red)
- Ice cream
- Mustard
- Sauces
- Savoury snacks
- Soups
- Soft drinks.

**E152** Black 7984 (Food Black 2, C.I. 27755) is a brown-to-black synthetic diazo food dye and usually comes as what chemists call a 'tetrasodium' salt. In addition to colouring foods, it is also found in some cosmetics. It appears to cause allergic or intolerance reactions, particularly amongst those with an aspirin intolerance.

Because of this, and the fact it is a histamine liberator that may worsen the symptoms of asthma, its use has been discontinued (delisted) in the USA and EU since 1984. It is also not permitted in Australia and Japan.

**E153** Vegetable carbon is a black/charcoal pigment that can increase hyperactivity in affected children and should be avoided by those with any allergies or intolerances. Whilst this black colouring can be obtained from various sources, including activated charcoal, blood, bones, meat, various fats, oils and resins or just the incomplete combustion of natural gas, it is normally derived from burnt vegetable matter. It is banned in the USA and only the vegetable-derived variety is permitted in Australia.

*Products that may contain E153*
- Jams
- Jellies
- Liquorice.

**E154** Brown FK (Kipper or Food Brown) is made from six azo dyes with sodium chloride and/or sodium sulphate. It is mainly used to give fish flesh a healthy pigment which will not leach or fade during cooking. It is banned in Austria, Australia, Japan, New Zealand, Switzerland, the USA and all EU countries except the UK.

*Products that may contain E154*

- Crisps
- Cooked meats, especially ham
- Cured and smoked fish, such as kippers and mackerel.

**E155** Brown HT is a brown azo dye used in chocolate cakes and biscuits. It can produce bad reactions in asthmatics and people who are allergic to aspirin and is known to induce skin sensitivity. It is thought to be a carcinogenic in food and to cause adverse reactions in children with ADHD. It is banned in Austria, Belgium, Denmark, France, Germany, Norway, Switzerland, Sweden and the USA.

**E160a** Carotenes – orange/yellow dyes - are available in both synthetic and natural forms but food manufacturers do not have to specify which one they use. Natural beta-carotene has been shown to be a powerful cancer preventive substance when ingested with natural vitamin E, vitamin C, selenium and zinc-rich foods. (Note: Do not take zinc sulphate as it has been shown to cause cancer.) On the other hand, synthetic beta-carotene has been shown to increase the risk of cancer and the death rate among smokers.

Even when beta-carotene is natural, the source is also important. Only purchase capsule and tablet supplements that list beta-carotene as natural and the source as *Dunaliella salina* algae or red palm on the label. (Almost all beta-carotene supplements do not specify the source of the beta-carotene.) Natural beta-carotene from carrots or carrot oil should be avoided as it is extracted with the extremely dangerous solvent hexane and hexane residue will always remain in the product. Hexane has been proven to cause birth defects, cancer and DNA damage. Ideally, natural beta-carotene (with the source given) should always contain natural vitamin E, which is a safe preservative. In cosmetics, it is labelled as C.I.75130.

**Note:** Cooked carrots are a rich source of beta-carotene. Try to buy only organic carrots as non-organic vegetables are heavily sprayed with pesticides. Fat or oil from avocado, coconut, fish, nuts, seeds etc should be eaten at the same time for the body to be able to absorb the beta-carotene and to process it into vitamin A. Natural beta-carotene cannot be converted into vitamin A in the body by diabetics, infants and people with gall bladder disorders or thyroid disorders.

**E160b** Annatto (Bixin, Norbixin) is a red colour; derived from a tree (*Bixa orellana*); water-soluble annatto contains bixin, a carotenoid, and the main colourant which may be interconverted by hydrolysis to norbixin. Annatto, bixin and norbixin can be used in a great variety of foods due to being either oil- or water-soluble. Annatto is known to cause urticaria (nettle rash) and flare-ups of angioneurotic oedema, also known as Quincke's oedema, which is the rapid oedema (swelling) of the deep layers of skin known as the dermis, subcutaneous tissue, mucosa and submucosal tissues.

Although similar to urticaria (hives), urticaria only occurs in the upper dermis. Annatto is also implicated in asthma (as it contains salicylic acid) and hyperactivity.

*Products that may contain E160b*

- Body paints
- Butter and margarine
- Cakes
- Cereals
- Cheese
- Coleslaw
- Cooking oils
- Crisps
- Custard
- Digestive aids
- Expectorant medicines
- Fabric dye
- Fish fingers
- Fruit and cream fillings and toppings
- Ice cream and ice lollies
- Icings
- Instant mashed potato
- Liqueurs
- Meatballs
- Mayonnaise
- Pastry
- Puddings
- Salad cream
- Sauces
- Smoked fish
- Snacks
- Soaps
- Soft drinks
- Spreads
- Textiles
- Varnishes
- Yoghurt.

**E161g** Canthaxanthin is a pink dye usually derived from beta-carotene and used to colour the skin in artificial suntan products where its use has given cause for concern due to eyesight problems, including deterioration in twilight vision, delays in adapting to the dark and sensitivity to glare. These products use greater quantities than are used in food and, although there is currently no direct evidence, the increasing use of canthaxanthin as a 'natural' substance in food is a cause for concern. It is banned in the USA.

*Products that may contain E161g*

- Chicken in breadcrumbs
- Confectionary and sweets
- Crab and lobster
- Fish fingers
- Farmed salmon and trout (to enhance the colour of the flesh)
- Egg yolks (it is included in feed for laying hens)
- Marshmallow biscuits
- Mushrooms
- Pickles
- Preserves
- Sauces.

**E170** Calcium carbonate (which is white) occurs naturally in chalk, coral, dolomite, eggshells (these consist of 94 per cent calcium carbonate), limestone, marble, pearls, stalactites, stalagmites and in the shells of many marine animals. It does not cause adverse effects at food additive levels but excessive consumption may cause bleeding anal fissures, constipation, flatulence and/or haemorrhoids. Because of its easy solubility, prolonged excessive consumption may result in high quantities in the blood, producing abdominal pain, confused behaviour, kidney or bladder stones and weak muscles.

*Products that may contain E170*
- Biscuits
- Bread
- Cakes
- Cleaning powders
- Confectionary and sweets
- Ice cream
- Tinned fruit and vegetables
- Toothpaste
- Vitamins and other supplements and medications
- White paint
- Wine.

**E173** Aluminium, as a food additive, is used for external decoration only – it can be found in the covering of dragées (bite-sized confectionery with a hard outer shell, such as 'silver balls' for decorating cakes) and is used to give a silvery finish to pills and tablets. It is also added to tap-water in some areas to remove discoloration and is widely used in antacid medicines. It can also be found in soft drinks in aluminium cans once past their sell-by dates, when the aluminium content of the drink has been found to exceed the limits laid down by the EU for drinking water, and the use of aluminium pots, pans and cooking utensils can also raise aluminium levels in cooking.

It has become apparent that an accumulation of aluminium in the cells of the nervous system can be toxic – it has been found in very high levels in the brain cells of individuals with Alzheimer's disease, accumulated in the neurofibrillary tangles and neuritic (senile) plaques that characterise the condition, but it is not yet known whether this is a cause or result of the disease. Several studies have also shown that excessive aluminium intake may have adverse effects on the metabolism of phosphorus and calcium in the human body and may induce or intensify skeletal abnormalities, such as osteoporosis. Increased urinary excretion of magnesium and calcium has been reported following regular antacid use.

**E180** Litholrubine BK is a reddish synthetic azo dye, used solely for colouring the rind of hard cheeses. Individuals with asthma, rhinitis or allergic skin problems may find their symptoms become worse following consumption of azo dyes. E180 is banned in Australia.

**E181** Tannic acid (tannins) is a brown dye and clarifying agent used in alcohol. It should be avoided by individuals with anaemia as it can hinder the absorption of iron and may cause migraines in susceptible individuals

# About the Author

Nat H Hawes SNHS Dip. (Advanced Nutrition and Sports Nutrition) has been studying and researching natural remedies, nutrients and the power of traditional foods and medicines since 2003. She believes, based on this research, that, unless nutrient deficiencies are tested for properly and shown to be present, extracted nutrient supplements are unnecessary and can do more harm than good. Natural and unrefined whole foods will provide the body with all the fuel it requires to function correctly and recover from most common ailments. She can be contacted through the following:

- Website: naturecures.co.uk
- Email: health@naturecures.co.uk
- Mobile: +44 (0)7966 519844